Kama Sutra

The Ultimate Sex Guide To Kama Sutra, Love Making and Sex Positions – Secret Techniques For Your Sex Life!

By: Rachel Hughes

Rachel Hughes

Disclaimer Notice:

Table of Contents

Rachel Hughes

Introduction

The Kama Sutra is an ancient text that has been around about 2,000 years. It would be foolish to believe that the book in its entirety, still rings true today. The Kama Sutra was one book in a group of books known as the Kama Shastra, though the Kama Sutra is the only one most of us are still familiar with. Although the book was written thousands of years ago, there are some aspects of the book that still pertain to modern, developed societies. Most of the book is based on love, desire, and relationships; only a small portion is attributed to sex positions. Although this is the case, many people still believe the Kama Sutra is mainly a book on sexual positioning and pleasure.

Coming to terms with the fact that sex and sexual fulfillment isn't just equated to penetrative sex is the first step in satisfying yourself and your partner. This book will take you in depth on different facets of the Kama Sutra and how they can create a more satisfying sex life for you and your partner. Along with various direct excerpts and quotations from the original, ancient Kama Sutra text by Vatsyayana, this book also has modern interpretations and practices commonly participated in by couples in today's society.

One thing to keep in mind when reading this book is that aside from some of the bizarre and almost comical parts (charms, recipes, and potions), there are a lot of aspects that are used in today's society and other developed worlds. It is interesting to see that populations over 2,000 years ago were still making love and performing oral sex and foreplay. Although women weren't seen as equals to men, in the bedroom they were highly respected and were to be made certain they were pleasured at the end of sexual intercourse.

I hope this book not only gives you insight into the past sexual practices that were spoken of and engaged in during ancient times as written in Kama Sutra text, but also shows you how much we relate to individuals who lived so long ago. This book will give you the tools you need to fulfill your sexual fantasies and desires along with a bunch of extra, historical information to share with your lover – maybe even practice?

Chapter 1
General Principles Of Kama Sutra

Kama Sutra is a well-known, historical guide to the principles of lovemaking, desire, sexual position and all around general sexual behaviors. This guide, though relatively dated, still applies to many facets of modern day sexual practices. Most of the Kama Sutra is dedicated to different principles and guidelines both male and female must abide by to have the most fulfilling sex life. There are also lots of talk and theory on the root of desire and passion. Some of the most common principles of Kama Sutra are still widely used today.

The Indians believe in following four most important principles of life to master your senses and achieve fulfillment in life and sexually. The four principles (or goals) are Dharma, Artha, Kama, and Moksha. Taken from the sacred texts of the original Kama Sutra by Vatsyayana, the four goals should be practiced as follows:

"Man, the period of whose life is one hundred years, should practice Dharma, Artha, and Kama at different times and in such a manner that they may harmonize together and not clash in any way. He should acquire learning in his childhood, in his youth and middle age he should attend to Artha and Kama, and in his old age, he should perform Dharma, and thus seek to gain Moksha, i.e. release from further transmigration. Or, on account of the uncertainty of life, he may practice them at times when they are enjoined to be practiced. But one thing is to be noted; he should lead the life of a religious student until he finishes his education.

Dharma is obedience to the command of the Shastra or Holy Writ of the Hindu's to do certain things, such as the performance of sacrifices, which are not generally done, because they do not belong to this world, and produce no visible effect; and not to do other things, such as eating meat, which is often done because it belongs to this world, and has visible effects. Dharma should be learned from the Shruti (Holy Writ), and from those conversant with it.

Artha is the acquisition of arts, land, gold, cattle, wealth, equipages and friends. It is, further, the protection of what is acquired, and the increase of what is protected. Artha should be learned from the king's officers, and from merchants who may be versed in the ways of commerce.

The Kama is the enjoyment of appropriate objects by the five senses of hearing, feeling, seeing, tasting and smelling, assisted by the mind together with the soul. The ingredient in this is a peculiar contact between the organ of sense and its object, and the consciousness of pleasure which arises from that contact is called The Kama. Kama is to be learned from the Kama Sutra (aphorisms on love) and the practice of citizens.

When all the three, viz. Dharma, Artha, and The Kama, come together, the former is better than the one which follows it, i.e. Dharma is better than Artha, and Artha is better than The Kama. But Artha should always be first practiced by the king for the livelihood of men is to be obtained from it only. Again, The Kama being the occupation of free women, they should prefer it to the other two, and these are exceptions to the general rule".

Translated to more modern terminology, Dharma is described as virtuous living. Whether these virtues are diving in origin or virtues that we have developed for ourselves is a matter of discussion. The definition of virtue is said to be the essence of our character and our morals or "the moral excellence of a person"; keeping to these morals every day equates to living virtuously. If you are religious, follow the holy virtues whereas individuals who aren't of religious backgrounds can develop morals of their own, usually relating to or in the attempt at moral excellence.

Artha pertains to the obtainment of material prosperity. For an individual to live and embrace the goal of Artha, they must seek to obtain wealth and many items others would see as wealthy. In modern day society, Artha could be seen as prosperity alone, not specified to material only. Individuals believe to be prosperous if they have a roof over their head, food in their fridge and bills paid. Prosperity can mean different things to different people because we all come from different backgrounds and upbringings. Living as if one is prosperous regarding attitude would put one far ahead of most humans today. In a world full of satisfaction, it would be wise to find prosperity in one's life outside of the shroud of material items.

The Kama is defined as "desire" and what we find desirable as human beings. What is interesting about Kama Sutra is that, historically, the desire was said to be something you can create and build on; not merely something that sparks when you meet a person. Kama Sutra described the difference between lust and desire, stating that we have the ability to create both. In modern times, we deem certain people to be desirable and cast out everyone else who doesn't have the particular features that we find helpful. This goes to show how over time, our view on love, desire, and lust has grown to be a bit shallower than previously intended.

This could be partly because there was a high amount of arranged marriages in ancient times so being able to make someone desirable to you out of necessity to reproduce would be a good trait to have. As time went on, arranged marriages in most developed worlds are seen as taboo and are no longer practiced. No arranged marriages mean the ability to choose, thus creating our vision of what we find desirable in a mate.

Moksha is liberation; freedom of ignorance. To follow Moksha, you need to seek wisdom and learn from everything you encounter. Strive for self-awareness, self-realization, and self-knowledge. Knowing who you are, what you stand for and what you want out of life falls into line with Moksha. A feeling of liberation and all-encompassing knowledge about who you are as an individual.

If one is unable to practice all of these at once, it is instructed that one should focus on living virtuously and being a good person before focusing on materialistic things and pleasure. According to Vatsyayana "A man practicing Dharma, Artha and Kama enjoy happiness now and in future. Any action which conduces to the practice of Dharma, Artha, and The Kama together, or of any two, or even one of them should be performed. But an action which conduces to the practice of one of them at the expense of the remaining two should not be performed."

There is a delicate balance when it comes to following Dharma, Artha, Kama and Moksha. According to Vatsyayana, the original

Kama Sutra author, there shouldn't be any conflict with practicing all of the goals, but if the conflict should arise, pleasure needs to focus on last. One of the biggest teachings this book is meant to educate individuals on is the importance that we as a person have on our lives. We create good days, and we create bad days; we are in control. Bettering oneself doesn't come easy and isn't something that happens overnight; certain aspects of life need to be learned through experience and mistakes.

The Kama Sutra knows the impact that common factors have on your sexual desire and drive. Someone who is stressed out, angry with themselves and unhappy is going to have a less than fulfilling sexual experience, regardless if they are with the person they love. Becoming aware of who we are as a person will have a profound effect on our ability to satisfy ourselves and our lover. Knowing yourself and loving yourself need to come first.

Chapter 2
Classifications And Love

The Kama Sutra states that there are several classifications of both men and women that are integral in the compatibility of couples. Both men and females are categorized into three different animals. The males are classified based on the length of their penis, and the women are classified by the depth of their vagina. The male classifications are: Shasha (hare), vrisha (bull), ashwas (horse), and the women are classified as mrigi (deer), vadavas (mare), hastinis (elephant).

For men, the classification components are as follows:

Shasha or hare-man, have an erection that is no longer than six finger breaths, or three inches in length when erect. It also describes his figure to be short but well-proportioned, and his penis is darker than the rest of his skin. His hair is also said to be silky and his teeth to be short and fine. He does not have a ravenous appetite for food, and he is a humble man with moderate carnal desires.

The vrisha or bull-man has a penis no longer than four inches in length when erect. He is said to be robust with a body like a tortoise with a hard belly and a fleshy chest. He has large eyes and a high forehead, the palms of his hands are pink, and he has a cruel and violent disposition.

The ashwas or horse-man has an erection around six inches long with a large framed body and a hard, muscular body. He desires his women to be hard and muscular as well as opposed to delicate; his knees are crooked, and he has very long extremities. He is known to be gluttonous, passionate, lazy and loves to sleep.

For women, the classification components are as follows:

The origin or deer woman has a vagina that is six fingers deep; she is a girly and delicate woman with a small head and perky breasts. Her legs are large and rounded, as are her arms. She has dark, curly hair and dark eyes and she tend to be jealous in nature. He vagina smells like a flower, her mind active and her demeanor is passionate when it comes to making love to her partner.

The vadavas or mare woman has a vagina that is nine fingers in depth. She has thick arms and broad shoulders and breasts. She is graceful in her walk and has a calm demeanor, dark eyes, long straight hair, and red hands and feet. Her vagina is said to smell of a lotus, and she has difficult reaching orgasm through penetrative sex.

The hastinis or elephant woman has a vagina that is twelve fingers in depth. She has large breasts, and a long nose, throat, and ears. She has yellow-tinged eyes and dark, long and thick hair while never thinking twice about committing a sin. She has long lips and a harsh voice while her hands and feet are short and fat. Her ejaculatory juices are abundant in nature and suffers from extreme gluttony while still being unable to achieve satisfaction in the bedroom.

The compatibility chart for each of these different classifications is as follows:

Equal pairs would be the hare and the deer, the bull and the mare, and the horse and the elephant. Unequal pairs would be hare and mare, hare and elephant, bull and deer, bull and elephant, horse and deer, horse and mare. The reason there are optimal compatibilities is that everyone is different and these certain classifications provide the ultimate pair. A short vagina and a long penis would have difficulty pleasuring one another because the penis would be painful for the women and the vagina would not be able to withstand deep penetration for the man.

It is common for women and men to contain several traits from one or more classifications; just like there is a wealth of continued knowledge on the topic. There is also classification based on stamina; the short timed, the moderate timed and the long timed. The man should also arouse the woman earlier because it takes women to climax. The Kama Sutra states that "by union with men, the lust, desire or passion of women is satisfied" and that women must reach climax before or during the climax of the male. The Kama Sutra describes four kinds of love

1) "Love resulting from constant and continual performance of love. In other words, love acquired by habit. Love resulting from the constant and continual performance of some act is called love acquired by constant practice and habit, as for instance the love of sexual intercourse, the love of hunting, the love of drinking, the love of gambling, etc., etc.

2) Love that comes from the imagination - love that proceeds from ideas, and emphasizes embracing, kissing, stroking, and scratching. Love which is felt for things to which we are not habituated, and which proceeds entirely from ideas, is called love resulting from imagination, as for instance that love which some men and women and eunuchs feel for the Auparishtaka or mouth congress, and that which is felt by all for such things as embracing, kissing, etc., etc.

3) Love that is mutual on both sides and has been proven to be true. The love which is mutual on both sides, and proved to

be true, when each looks upon the other as his or her very own, such is called love resulting from belief by the learned."

4) Love resulting from experience - love that is known only to others because it is never analyzed as such (and is, therefore, the superior form of love). In the Kama Sutra, the love resulting from the perception of external objects is quite evident and well known to the world. Because the pleasure which it affords is superior to the pleasure of the other kinds of love, which exists only for its sake."

In the Kama Sutra, the love resulting from the perception of external objects is quite evident and well known to the world. Because the pleasure which it affords is superior to the pleasure of the other kinds of love, which exists only for its sake.

Love is also constituted as an art form and with such, the following 64 arts (according to the Kama Sutra) need to be studied to understand the art of love. The following 64 studies are taken directly from the original Kama Sutra:

- "Singing

- Playing on musical instruments

- Dancing

- Union of dancing, singing, and playing instrumental music

- Writing and drawing

- Tattooing

- Arraying and adorning an idol with rice and flowers

- Spreading and arranging beds or couches of flowers, or flowers upon the ground

- Coloring the teeth, garments, hair, nails and bodies, i.e. staining, dyeing, coloring and painting the same

- Fixing stained glass into a floor

- The art of making beds, and spreading out carpets and cushions for reclining

- Playing on musical glasses filled with water

- Storing and accumulating water in aqueducts, cisterns, and reservoirs

- Picture making, trimming and decorating

- Stringing of rosaries, necklaces, garlands and wreaths

- Binding of turbans and chaplets, and making crests and top-knots of flowers

- Scenic representations, stage playing Art of making ear ornaments Art

- Preparing perfumes and odors

- Proper disposition of jewels and decorations, and adornment in dress

- Magic or sorcery

- Quickness of hand or manual skill

- Culinary art, i.e. cooking and cookery

- Making lemonades, sherbets, acidulated drinks, and spirituous extracts with proper flavor and color

- Tailor's work and sewing

- Making parrots, flowers, tufts, tassels, bunches, bosses, knobs, etc., out of yarn or thread

- Solution of riddles, enigmas, covert speeches, verbal puzzles and enigmatical questions

- A game, which consisted in repeating verses, and as one person finished, another person had to commence at once, repeating another verse, beginning with the same letter with which the last speaker's verse ended, whoever failed to repeat was considered to have lost, and to be subject to pay a forfeit or stake of some kind

- The art of mimicry or imitation

- Reading, including chanting and intoning

- Study of sentences difficult to pronounce. It is played as a game chiefly by women, and children and consists of a difficult sentence being given, and when repeated quickly, the words are often transposed or badly pronounced

- Practice with sword, single stick, quarter staff and bow and arrow

- Drawing inferences, reasoning or inferring

- Carpentry, or the work of a carpenter

- Architecture, or the art of building

- Knowledge about gold and silver coins, and jewels and gems

- Chemistry and mineralogy

- Colouring jewels, gems, and beads

- Knowledge of mines and quarries

- Gardening; knowledge of treating the diseases of trees and plants, of nourishing them, and determining their ages

- Art of cock fighting, quail fighting and ram fighting

- Art of teaching parrots and starlings to speak

- Art of applying perfumed ointments to the body, and of dressing the hair with unguents and perfumes and braiding it

- The art of understanding writing in cipher, and the writing of words in a peculiar way

- The art of speaking by changing the forms of words. It is of various kinds. Some speak by changing the beginning and end of words, others by adding unnecessary letters between every syllable of a word, and so on

- Knowledge of language and the vernacular dialects

- Art of making flower carriages

- Art of framing mystical diagrams, of addressing spells and charms, and binding armlets

- Mental exercises, such as completing stanzas or verses on receiving a part of them; or supplying one, two or three lines when the remaining lines are given indiscriminately from different verses, so as to make the whole an entire verse concerning its meaning; or arranging the words of a verse written irregularly by separating the vowels from the consonants, or leaving them out altogether; or putting into verse or prose sentences represented by signs or symbols. There are many other such exercises.

- Composing poems

- Knowledge of dictionaries and vocabularies

- Knowledge of ways of changing and disguising the appearance of persons

- Knowledge of the art of changing the appearance of things, such as making cotton appear as silk, coarse and common things to appear as fine and good.

- Various ways of gambling

- Art of obtaining possession of the property of others using mantras or incantations

- Skill in youthful sports

- Knowledge of the rules of society, and of how to pay respect and compliments to others

- Knowledge of the art of war, of arms, of armies, etc.

- Knowledge of gymnastics

- Art of knowing the character of a man from his features

- Knowledge of scanning or constructing verses

- Arithmetical recreations

- Making artificial flowers

- Making figures and images in clay."

It is said that a man who engages in these different types of arts can win over the heart of women whereas a man who doesn't will have a difficult time winning over a woman's heart. This is a lot to expect from a man, and this certainly doesn't reflect the views of modern day society, however, historically in Indian practice, this was expected of men who wanted to gain a satisfying sex life.

There are also many reasons a woman may reject a man, many of which are outlined in the Kama Sutra. According to the Kama Sutra, men that are rejected by women usually

"Affection for her husband

Desire of lawful progeny

Want of opportunity

Anger at being addressed by the man too familiarly

Difference in rank of life

Want of certainty on account of the man being devoted traveling

Thinking that the man may be attached to some other person

Fear of the man's not keeping his intentions secret

Thinking that the man is too devoted to his friends, and has too great a regard for them

The apprehension that he is not in earnest

Bashfulness on account of his being an illustrious man

Fear on account of his being powerful, or possessed of too impetuous passion, in the case of the deer woman

Bashfulness on account of his being too clever

The thought of having once lived with him on friendly terms only

Contempt of his want of knowledge of the world

Distrust of his low character

Disgust at his want of perception of her love for him

In the case of an elephant woman, the thought that he is a hare man or a man of weak passion

Compassion lest anything should befall him on account of his passion

Despair at her imperfections

Fear of discovery

Disillusion at seeing his gray hair or shabby appearance

Fear that he may be employed by her husband to test her chastity

The thought that he has too much regard for morality."

One thing that can be agreed upon in modern day belief is that love can change your life. Love is a necessity for the well-being of our individuality and overall self. Living a loveless life would be one of loneliness and unhappiness. Kama Sutra attempts to prevent people from living loveless lives by telling us how to get the attention of other human beings. As far as the beliefs nowadays, to win over the heart of someone else, you need to both communicate what you are looking for in a relationship. Expressing your likes and dislikes will give each other a better idea of personality and what would make the other happy.

Communication in a relationship is something that cannot be stressed enough. You can't expect to fall in love with someone if you never communicate with them, and vice versa. You both need to be comfortable expressing emotions with one another or love will never be one of the emotions you both experience. Lust can be felt by looking at one another; love can be felt by speaking with one another.

Chapter 3
Behavior Inside And Outside The Bedroom

In order to have a fulfilling sex life, you have to have an individual behavior both inside and outside the bedroom. The Kama Sutra states different ways in which men and women must act; we will get into those later. Starting off, though, behavior inside and outside the bedroom are rarely ever comparable, but they do work interdependently. For example, going on a few dates with an individual you think is attractive but you have yet to be able to carry on a conversation without being put off by something your date says. This same date tends to be angry and mean to other people, sometimes at you as well. You both start drinking and things start to heat up, and it turns out that your date is a very passionate lover but not a very personable person. This may be a turn off to some people.

Both your behavior towards your lover inside and outside the bedroom will reflect your overall compatibility with one another. As far as behavior inside the bedroom, Kama Sutra state there are certain ways in which a man and a woman should behave towards one another before taking each other to bed. According to the Kama Sutra, "The man who is ingenious and wise, who is accompanied by a friend, and who knows the intentions of others, as also the proper time and place for doing everything, can gain over, very easily, even a woman who is very hard to be obtained." There are also certain kinds of women that men should avoid; according to the Kama Sutra. These can all be interpreted different ways in modern day. These types of women include:

- A leper; probably due to disease and ill health. Leprosy was a dangerous and contagious disease in those times. The thought of contracting such a debilitating and deforming disease was terrifying.

- A lunatic; no one wants to be with someone "loony". Lunatics can be a danger to themselves, their lovers and their family members.

- A woman turned out of caste; back when the caste system was a huge determining social factor. Now, this would equate to a celebrity dating a blue collar worker of a wealthy man dating a poor woman.

- A woman who reveals secrets; this was meant to avoid any woman who couldn't be trusted. Confidence is an important trait in relationships and is necessary to sustain a relationship.

- A woman who publicly expresses desire for sexual intercourse; this could be a turn off to men because it may be a red flag that she could sleep around or perhaps engage in infidelity. In those times, men were allowed to sleep around a bit more than women were.

- A woman who is extremely white; Paleness could be an indicator of someone who never leaves the house or is ill in some way.

- A woman who is extremely black; This was back when racism and slavery were highly prominent.

- A bad-smelling woman; someone who smells bad equates to someone with poor hygiene. Having proper hygiene is important to stay healthy and make yourself desirable. A woman with bad hygiene could be seen as lazy o someone who just doesn't care.

- A woman who is a near relation; such as a cousin or a niece/nephew. Incest was (and still is) frowned upon ethically and health-wise. When families begin to reproduce within their gene pool, mutations begin to occur.

- A woman who is a female friend; it may be hard to break past the friend feeling. To avoid this difficulty, women who are your friend should not be considered for lovers.

- A woman who leads the life of an ascetic; this would mean someone who does not do anything for pleasure; no sex, kissing, embrace, love. For obvious reasons, the Kama Sutra recommends avoiding this type of woman.

- And, lastly the wife of a relation, of a friend, of a learned Brahman, and of the king.

Although there are many types of women the Kama Sutra states to avoid; there isn't much emphasis on the types of men that women should avoid. I think that a lot of the same statements can be echoed for men as well. One trait that wasn't discussed was physical abuse. No abuse of any kind should occur in any form from either the male or the female. If abuse of any kind occurs, the relationship should be ended immediately.

During sex, the Kama Sutra describes sex as being comparable to combat. When men and women get into the passion of sexual intercourse, they can instinctually strike out at one another in passion. The Kama Sutra describes several types of hits and blows, all of which are not done out of malice, only out of passion.

The most common places for individuals to strike out at one another is:

- The shoulders

- The head

- The space between the breasts

- The back

- The middle part of the body

- The sides

There are four different types of strikes:

- Striking with the back of the hand

- Striking with the fingers a little contracted

- Striking with the fist

- Striking with the open palm of the hand

The Kama Sutra also analyzes the sounds made during hitting and sexual intercourse. The sounds are all based on the force of the hit and the area in which the hit was inflicted. The sounds and cries that come from the individual are also listed among the sounds heard.

According to the Kama Sutra:

- "The sound Hin

- The thundering sound

- The cooing sound

- The weeping sound

- The sound Phut

- The sound Phât

- The sound Sût

- The sound Plât"

Besides these, there are also words having a meaning, such as 'mother', and those that are expressive of prohibition, sufficiency, desire of liberation, pain or praise, and to which may be added sounds like those of the dove, the cuckoo, the green pigeon, the parrot, the bee, the sparrow, the flamingo, the duck, and the quail, which are all occasionally made use of.

Blows with the fist should be given on the back of the woman while she is sitting on the lap of the man, and she should give blows in return, abusing the man as if she were angry, and making the cooing and the weeping sounds. While the woman is engaged in Congress, the space between the breasts should be struck with the back of the hand, slowly at first, and then proportionately to the increasing excitement, until the end.

At this time the sounds Hin and others may be made, alternately or optionally, according to habit. When the man, making the sound Phât, strikes the woman on the head, with the fingers of his hand a little contracted, it is called Prasritaka, which means striking with the fingers of the hand a little contracted. In this case, the appropriate sounds are the cooing sound, the sound Phât and the sound Phut in the interior of the mouth, and at the end of Congress the sighing and weeping sounds.

The sound Phât is an imitation of the sound of a bamboo being split, while the sound Phut is like the sound made by something falling into the water.

At all times when kissing and such like things are begun, the woman should give a reply with a hissing sound. During the excitement when the woman is not accustomed to striking, she continually utters words expressive of prohibition, sufficiently, or desire of liberation, as well as the words 'father', 'mother', intermingled with the sighing, weeping and thundering sounds. 1 Towards the conclusion of the Congress, the breasts, the jaghana, and the sides of the woman should be pressed with the open palms of the hand, with some force, until the end of it, and then sounds like those of the quail or the goose should be made.

'The characteristics of manhood are said to consist of roughness and impetuosity, while weakness, tenderness, sensibility, and an inclination to turn away from unpleasant things are the distinguishing marks of womanhood. The excitement of passion and peculiarities of habit may sometimes cause contrary results to appear, but these do not last long, and in the end, the natural state is resumed.'

The wedge on the bosom, the scissors on the head, the piercing instrument on the cheeks, and the pinchers on the breasts and sides, may also be taken into consideration with the other four modes of striking, and thus give eight ways altogether. But these four ways of striking with instruments are peculiar to the people of the southern countries, and the marks caused by them are seen on the breasts of their women. They are local peculiarities, but Vatsyayana is of opinion that the practice of them is painful, barbarous, and base, and quite unworthy of imitation.

In the same way, anything that is a local peculiarity should not always be adopted elsewhere, and even in the place where the practice is prevalent, excess of it should always be avoided. Instances of the dangerous use of them may be given as follows. The king of the Panchalas killed the courtesan Madhavasena by means of the wedge during the congress. King Satakarni Satavahana of the Kuntalas deprived his great Queen Malayavati of her life by a pair of scissors, and Naradeva, whose hand was deformed, blinded a dancing girl by directing a piercing instrument in a wrong way. 'About these things, there cannot be either enumeration or any definite rule. Congress having once commenced, passion alone gives birth to all the acts of the parties.'

'Such passionate actions and amorous gesticulations or movements, which arise on the spur of the moment, and during sexual intercourse, cannot be defined, and are as irregular as dreams. A horse having once attained the fifth degree of motion goes on with blind speed, regardless of pits, ditches, and posts in his way; and in the same manner a loving pair become blind with passion in the heat of congress, and go on with great impetuosity, paying not the least regard to excess.

For this reason, one who is well acquainted with the science of love, and knowing his strength, as also the tenderness, impetuosity, and strength of the young women should act accordingly. The various modes of enjoyment are not for all times or all persons, but they should only be used at the proper time. And in the proper countries and places," as quoted directly from the Kama Sutra.

Rachel Hughes

Chapter 4
Kissing Techniques

Kissing is one of the most intimate practices we share with one another. One of the reasons there are so many different kissing techniques is because kissing can be the key to arousal for nearly every individual. Your lips contain some of the highest concentrations of nerves. Kama Sutra has an abundance of kisses, biting and nibbling techniques that need to be shared.

According to the Kama Sutra, "Kissing is of four kinds in Kama Sutra: moderate, contracted, pressed, and soft, according to the different parts of the body which are kissed, for different kinds of kisses are appropriate for different parts of the body."

Askew kiss: When the heads of the two are tilted in opposite directions, pressing their lips together in a kiss. This kiss is most commonly seen in movies because the different direction allows you to see the kiss more clearly. This is an incredibly intimate kiss and is often the initiation of a sexual encounter. This is also one of the most popular kisses because of your ability to penetrate deeper with your tongue along with better contact between the lips of both lovers.

Bent kiss: When one of the two throws his head back and the other holding it over her chin and kisses him. This kiss allows for a great deal of affection and tenderness. This kiss is commonly seen when the male is making love from the front (missionary position) and the woman throws her head back in euphoria. As she throws her head back, he kisses her lips. This kiss is incredible sensual and sweet.

Direct kiss: When the lips of both bind directly and suck as if it were a ripe fruit or as if sucking on your skin to get off a piece of chocolate. This kiss can be incorporated with nibbling, caressing, and sucking on the lips individually to add a bit more excitement. These kisses can be done for a long period of time, making them more passionate than other kisses.

Kiss pressure: The lips are pressed tightly with your mouth closed. These kisses are also known as "pecks". They are done quickly and not meant for a long period of contact. These kisses are usually done at the beginning of relationships, when you are just getting to know one another or as a quick good morning or goodbye kiss. These kisses can also incorporate biting, making it a bit more aggressive. The biting should not be done for an extended period of time to avoid injury or discomfort.

Top kiss: When one partner sucks on the upper lip and the other sucks on the bottom lip. This is an incredibly sensual and romantic kiss, usually used as a seduction technique. Switching between to two kisses using your tongue makes the kiss even more erotic and exciting.

Kiss clip: This is done when one of the partners uses their tongue to touch their lover's teeth, tongue, lips, etc. This is said to be the initiation for the "fight of the tongues" which can be erotic and exciting for both involved parties. Some lovers prefer not to use tongue as much as other individual's do; this kiss will confirm if your lover likes to kiss with tongue or not.

Throbbing kiss: When one of the lovers keeps their mouth closed or slightly open, while the other one kisses then tenderly all over their upper and bottom lips, moving to the corners of their mouth. These kisses are highly sensuous and provide a great deal of intimacy when done with a lover.

Contact Kiss: This is done after sexual tension and desire have built to unbearable amounts. This kiss is when one of the lovers lightly touches the others mouth with theirs, creating an almost cringe worthy sexual tension. The contact is meant to be done lightly but with high intensity.

Kiss to ignite the flame is a kiss that is done in the corner of the mouth. This kiss is meant to leave the other wanting more. This kiss can be done after a date or at the beginning of a sexual encounter. This kiss can also be used for teasing.

Kiss to distract is done, usually by the woman, to distract the other partner from their current distraction. This kiss is done in movies when something needs to be done by someone else so the woman grabs the males face and pulls it to hears, kissing him passionately and forcefully. This kiss is also meant to grace other areas of the body as well such as the neck, arms, chest, genitals, thighs, legs, butt, nipples, etc.

Nominal or farewell kiss: When you kiss your lovers mouth, then place two fingers on their lips afterwards. A quiet yet sensual farewell at the end of a date or before a trip.

Eyelash kiss (also known as butterfly kisses): When you flutter your eye lashes against the skin of your lover, usually around the lips, cheeks, forehead, nose and ears. This kiss is done using your eye lashes to gently brush against your lover's skin as you blink quickly or flutter your eyes.

Kiss with a finger is done when one of the lovers puts a single finger in the others mouth, letting them suck on it for a second before removing it and brushing it over their lips. This kiss is done as a prelude to oral sex due to its inviting and seductive nature.

Kiss with two fingers: When one lover places two fingers in their mouth and then presses them against the lips of their lover. This kiss is meant to be erotic and be a precursor for oral sex.

Kiss that awakens: This kiss is used for just that, to awaken. While the lover is sleeping, this kiss is done on the sleeping lovers temples or forehead to wake them tenderly. This affectionate kiss can be done prior to sexual intercourse or if the lover needs to be awakened for the day's duties.

Public kiss is done in public and is meant to show the world how you feel about one another. This kiss isn't meant to be a passionate embrace with a long lasting kiss, only as a soft kiss on either the neck, hand or face. This kiss is done in public to show the respect and admiration you have for one another.

Per the Kama Sutra, "There is also a fifth kind of kiss called the 'greatly pressed kiss', which is effected by taking hold of the lower lip between two fingers, and then, after touching it with the tongue, pressing it with great force with the lip. There are a variety of other kisses couples can incorporate into their relationship. The Kama Sutra states below, another several kissing techniques.

"When a man kisses the upper lip of a woman, while she in return kisses his lower lip, it is called the 'kiss of the upper lip'

When one of them takes both the lips of the other between his or her own, it is called 'a clasping kiss'. A woman, however, only takes this kind of kiss from a man who has no moustache. And on the occasion of this kiss, if one of them touches the teeth, the tongue, and the palate of the other, with his or her tongue, it is called the 'fighting of the tongue'. In the same way, the pressing of the teeth of the one against the mouth of the other is to be practiced.

When a woman looks at the face of her lover while he is asleep and kisses it to show her intention or desire, it is called a 'kiss that kindles love'.

When a woman kisses her lover while he is engaged in business, or while he is quarrelling with her, or while he is looking at something else, so that his mind may be turned away, it is called a 'kiss that turns away'.

When a lover coming home late at night kisses his beloved, who is asleep on her bed, in order to show her his desire, it is called a 'kiss that awakens'. On such an occasion the woman may pretend to be asleep at the time of her lover's arrival, so that she may know his intention and obtain respect from him.

When a person kisses the reflection of the person he loves in a mirror, in water, or on a wall, it is called a 'kiss showing the intention'. When a person kisses a child sitting on his lap, or a picture, or an image, or figure, in the presence of the person beloved by him, it is called a 'transferred kiss'.

When at night at a theatre, or in an assembly of caste men, a man coming up to a woman kisses a finger of her hand if she be standing, or a toe of her foot if she be sitting, or when a woman is shampooing her lover's body, places her face on his thigh (as if she was sleepy) so as to inflame his passion, and kisses his thigh or great toe, it is called a 'demonstrative kiss'."

With kissing there also comes to aspect of biting. Biting is highly erotic and sensual and is done by a vast majority of couples in the bedroom. The Kama Sutra states the different types of bites that exist and their relevance in sexual encounters. The body has multiple pressure points and pleasure points, these are targeted when biting and kissing is being done.

It is said by some that there is no fixed time or order between the embrace, the kiss, and the pressing or scratching with the nails or fingers, but that all these things should be done generally before sexual union takes place, while striking and making the various sounds generally takes place at the time of the union. Vatsyayana, however, thinks that anything may take place at any time, for love does not care for time or order

On the occasion of the first congress, kissing and the other things mentioned above should be done moderately, they should not be continued for a long time, and should be done alternately. On subsequent occasions, however, the reverse of all this may take place, and moderation will not be necessary, they may continue for a long time, and, for the purpose of kindling love, they may be all done at the same time."

When two lovers are writhing in passion, it isn't uncommon for them to incorporate other forms of intimacy such as using their nails and biting and sometimes striking out at one another, gently of course. According to the Kama Sutra, there are certain occasions when scratching or pressing your nails against your loved one is practiced. These four different occasions are: on the first visit, at the time of setting out on a journey (traveling or exploration), on the return from the journey, when the lover is angry with the other lover and there is a reconciliation, and then the woman lover is inebriated.

The intensity surrounding each of these occasions is what makes the use of nails so common. Nail biting it commonly incorporated with biting, not simply done on its own. Due to the aggressive nature of using nails and teeth, it is only practiced when both parties are in agreement of its use. There are eight different kinds of nail presses the produce eight different markings, through which their names were created. The following markings are as follows:

- Sounding

- Half moon

- A circle

- A line

- A tiger's nail or claw

- A peacock's foot

- The jump of a hare

- The leaf of a blue lotus

Like everything in the Kama Sutra, the nails were also placed into a classification. Everyone's nails are different therefore some individuals will be able to produce nail markings that other individuals may not be capable of. Due to this, the ancient text described three different types of nails with which you could classify yourself in. The three kinds are small, middling and large. The nails are supposed to be clea, bright, convex, soft, glossy in appearance and well set. There should be no nails missing, all ten nails should be present.

According to the Kama Sutra:

"Large nails, which give grace to the hands, and attract the hearts of women from their appearance, are possessed by the

Bengalese. Small nails, which can be used in various ways, and are to be applied only with the object of giving pleasure, are possessed by the people of the southern districts. Middling nails, which contain the properties of both the above kinds, belong to the people of the Maharashtra.

When a person presses the chin, the breasts, the lower lip, or the jaghana of another so softly that no scratch or mark is left, but only the hair on the body becomes erect from the touch of the nails, and the nails themselves make a sound, it is called a 'sounding or pressing with the nails'. This pressing is used in the case of a young girl when her lover shampoos her, scratches her head, and wants to trouble or frighten her.

The curved mark with the nails, which is impressed on the neck and the breasts, is called the 'half-moon'.

When the half-moons are impressed opposite to each other, it is called a 'circle'. This mark with the nails is generally made on the navel, the small cavities about the buttocks, and on the joints of the thigh.

A mark in the form of a small line, and which can be made on any part of the body, is called a 'line'.

This same line, when it is curved, and made on the breast, is called a 'tiger's nail'.

When a curved mark is made on the breast by means of the five nails, it is called a 'peacock's foot'. This mark is made with the object of being praised, for it requires a great deal of skill to make it properly.

When five marks with the nails are made close to one another near the nipple of the breast, it is called 'the jump of a hare'.

A mark made on the breast or on the hips in the form of a leaf of the blue lotus is called the 'leaf of a blue lotus'.

When a person is going on a journey, and makes a mark on the thighs, or on the breast, it is called a 'token of remembrance'. On such an occasion three or four lines are impressed close to one another with the nails.

Here ends the marking with the nails. Marks of other kinds than the above may also be made with the nails, for the ancient authors say that, as there are innumerable degrees of skill among men (the practice of this art being known to all), so there are innumerable ways of making these marks. And as pressing or marking with the nails is independent of love, no one can say with certainty how many different kinds of marks with the nails do actually exist."

Vatsyayana says, "that as variety is necessary in love, so love is to be Produced by means of variety. It is on this account that courtesans, who are well acquainted with various ways and means, become so desirable, for if variety is sought in all the arts and amusements, such as archery and others, how much more should it be sought after in the present case. The marks of the nails should not be made on married women, but particular kinds of marks may be made on their private parts for the remembrance and increase of love."

Several direct quotes from Kama Sutra in regards to nail pressing and digging are as follows:

"The love of a woman who sees the marks of nails on the private parts of her body, even though they are old and almost worn out, becomes again fresh and new. If there be no marks of nails to remind a person of the passages of love, then love is lessened in the same way as when no union takes place for a long time."

"Even when a stranger sees at a distance a young woman with the marks of nails on her breast, he is filled with love and respect for her."

"A man, also, who carries the marks of nails and teeth on some parts of his body, influences the mind of a woman, even though it be ever so firm. In short, nothing tends to increase love so much as the effects of marking with the nails, and biting."

The Kama Sutra also has various opinions on the scope of biting. Biting is common among couples and as stated before, goes hand in hand with the use of nail pressing and scratching. The Kama Sutra recommends teeth be white, equal, unbroken and with sharp ends. There is much emphasis on proportion in the Kama Sutra, the teeth are no exception. The different types of bites are as follows:

- The hidden bite

- The swollen bite

- The point

- The line of points

- The coral and the jewel

- The line of jewels

- The broken cloud

- The biting of the boar

The hidden bite is a bite that, when done correctly, is only noticeable by localized redness on the skin. The bite leaves no indentations, bruising or marks of any kind – only redness.

The swollen bite is when both sides of the skin are bitten down on at the same time. Almost as if you were pinching a pimple with your teeth, except a larger amount of skin is taken between the teeth. Left behind are the indentations of the teeth on either end of the skin.

When two teeth are used to bite a small portion of the skin, this bite is called the "point". This is a simple, easy to do bite that involves almost pinching the skin with your teeth.

In order to perform the bite 'line of points," you need to bite down or press down on the skin with your mouth, leaving indents in a line. The portions of the skin are small and not highly noticeable; a common fear of people whom must maintain a strict dress code.

The coral and the jewel bite is done when both the lips and teeth are used. Wth your mouth slightly open, come down on the skin, pressing firmly and sucking in slightly to have your lips leave marks on the skin. The coral is the lip and the teeth are the jewels, equating to the name "coral and the jewel".

Using all of your teeth to bite down in a single area of the skin will create a line of indentations where your teeth were lined. This jewels are supposed to be each individual indentation so depending on how wide you open your mouth and bite; you are looking at around 6-8 teeth marks for your upper teeth.

A popular bite that is meant for the breast is a bite called the "broken cloud". This bite is a series of indentations from biting in uneven rows, consecutively around one another. The bites are done almost as if you were drawing a cloud with your teeth but never connected the rows.

The biting of the boar is a bunch of broad rows of bites – as if a boar was biting at your skin. These bites are performed on the breasts and the shoulders and should be done carefully to not break the skin.

According to the Kama Sutra:

"The lower lip is the place on which the 'hidden bite', the swollen bite', and the 'point' are made; again the 'swollen bite' and the 'coral and the jewel' bite are done on the cheek. Kissing, pressing with the nails, and biting are the ornaments of the left cheek, and when the word cheek is used it is to be understood as the left cheek.

Both the 'line of points' and the 'line of jewels' are to be impressed on the throat, the arm pit, and the joints of the thighs; but the 'line of points' alone is to be impressed on the forehead and the thighs.

'When a man bites a woman forcibly, she should angrily do the same to him with double force. Thus a "point" should be returned with a "line of points", and a "line of points" with a "broken cloud", and if she be excessively chafed, she should at once begin a love quarrel with him.

At such a time she should take hold of her lover by the hair, and bend his head down, and kiss his lower lip, and then, being intoxicated with love, she should shut her eyes and bite him in various places. Even by day, and in a place of public resort, when her lover shows her any mark that she may have inflicted on his body, she should smile at the sight of it, and turning her face as if she were going to chide him, she should show him with an angry look the marks on her own body that have been made by him. Thus if men and women act according to each other's liking, their love for each other will not be lessened even in one hundred years."

Chapter 5
Oral Sex And Foreplay

When it comes to oral sex and foreplay, the Kama Sutra has a lot of different recommendations and ideas. A lot of these ideas – most of them in fact, are used by couples regularly. Starting with foreplay, this is a commonly overlooked part of love making. A lot of the time, foreplay is ignored by both parties because of the time it takes and the belief that actual intercourse feels better than foreplay. For people who actively participate in foreplay, most will tell you that it is their favorite part. A lot of men (and women for that matter) don't realize that women have a difficult time reaching orgasm during penetrative sex without foreplay or other forms of clitoral stimulation.

Because of the amount of time it takes a woman to reach orgasm, foreplay is recommended before each sexual encounter. The clitoris on the women needs to be stimulated before and during sex in order for her to reach climax. Everyone is different but for the majority of women, this is the case. Foreplay can involve a large variety of technique, oral pleasure, toys and other aphrodisiacs. Generally, foreplay is started off by kissing, slowly undressing and embracing one another. Foreplay can also involve sweet talking, dirty talking, watching pornography and lightly touching one another through the clothes.

Once undressed, foreplay will move to involve either the fingering, licking and sucking of the vagina along with sucking and licking of the penis. Kissing, touching and stroking is the main goal of foreplay, as is arousal. Extra focus needs to be placed on the women's clitoris in order for her to climax around the same time as the male.

Oral sex has several different techniques, the ancient text of Kama Sutra goes over several different oral techniques for both the male and the female. Oral sex, according to the Kama Sutra, is done one of the following ways:

"THERE are two kinds of eunuchs, those that are disguised as males, and those that are disguised as females. Eunuchs disguised as females imitate their dress, speech, gestures, tenderness, timidity, simplicity, softness and bashfulness. The acts that are done on the jaghana or middle parts of women, are done in the mouths of these eunuchs, and this is called Auparishtaka. 1 These eunuchs derive their imaginable pleasure, and their livelihood from this kind of congress, and they lead the life of courtesans. So much concerning eunuchs disguised as females.

Eunuchs disguised as males keep their desires secret, and when they wish to do anything they lead the life of shampooers. Under the pretence of shampooing, a eunuch of this kind embraces and draws towards himself the thighs of the man whom he is shampooing, and after this he touches the joints of his thighs and his jaghana, or central portions of his body. Then, if he finds the lingam of the man erect, he presses it with his hands and chaffs him for getting into that state. If after this, and after knowing his intention, the man does not tell the eunuch to proceed, then the latter does it of his own accord and begins the congress. If however he is ordered by the man to do it, then he disputes with him, and only consents at last with difficulty.

The following eight things are then done by the eunuch one after the other:

- The nominal congress

- Biting the sides

- Pressing outside

- Pressing inside

- Kissing

- Rubbing

- Sucking a mango fruit

- Swallowing up

At the end of each of these, the eunuch expresses his wish to stop, but when one of them is finished, the man desires him to do another, and after that is done, then the one that follows it, and so on.

When, holding the man's lingam with his hand, and placing it between his lips, the eunuch moves about his mouth, it is called the 'nominal congress'.

When, covering the end of the lingam with his fingers collected together like the bud of a plant or flower, the eunuch presses the sides of it with his lips, using his teeth also, it is called 'biting the sides'.

When, being desired to proceed, the eunuch presses the end of the lingam with his lips closed together, and kisses it as if he were drawing it out, it is called the 'outside pressing'.

When, being asked to go on, he puts the lingam further into his mouth, and presses it with his lips and then takes it out, it is called the 'inside pressing'.

When, holding the lingam in his hand, the eunuch kisses it as if he were kissing the lower lip, it is called 'kissing'.

When, after kissing it, he touches it with his tongue everywhere, and passes the tongue over the end of it, it is called 'rubbing'.

When, in the same way, he puts the half of it into his mouth, and forcibly kisses and sucks it, this is called 'sucking a mango fruit'.

And lastly, when, with the consent of the man, the eunuch puts the whole lingam into his mouth, and presses it to the very end, as if he were going to swallow it up, it is called 'swallowing up'.

Striking, scratching, and other things may also be done during this kind of congress.

The Auparishtaka is practiced also by unchaste and wanton women, female attendants and serving maids, i.e. those who are not married to anybody, but who live by shampooing.

The Acharyas (i.e. ancient and venerable authors) are of opinion that this Auparishtaka is the work of a dog and not of a man, because it is a low practice, and opposed to the orders of the Holy Writ, and because the man himself suffers by bringing his lingam into contact with the mouths of eunuchs and women. But Vatsyayana says that the orders of the Holy Writ do not affect those who resort to courtesans, and the law prohibits the practice of the Auparishtaka with married women only. As regards the injury to the male, that can be easily remedied.

The people of Eastern India do not resort to women who practice the Auparishtaka.

The people of Ahichhatra resort to such women, but do nothing with them, so far as the mouth is concerned.

The people of Saketa do with these women every kind of mouth congress, while the people of Nagara do not practice this, but do every other thing.

The people of the Shurasena country, on the southern bank of the Jumna, do everything without any hesitation, for they say that women being naturally unclean, no one can be certain about their character, their purity, their conduct, their practices, their confidences, or their speech. They are not however on this account to be abandoned, because religious law, on the authority of which they are reckoned pure, lays down that the udder of a cow is clean at the time of milking, though the mouth of a cow, and also the mouth of her calf, are considered unclean by the Hindoos. Again a dog is clean when he seizes a deer in hunting, though food touched by a dog is otherwise considered very unclean. A bird is clean when it causes a fruit to fall from a tree by pecking at it, though things eaten by crows and other birds are considered unclean. And the mouth of a woman is clean for kissing and such like things at the time of sexual intercourse. Vatsyayana moreover thinks that in all these things connected with love, everybody should act according to the custom of his country, and his own inclination.

There are also the following verses on the subject:

'The male servants of some men carry on the mouth congress with their masters. It is also practiced by some citizens, who know each other well, among themselves. Some women of the harem, when they are amorous, do the acts of the mouth on the yonis of one another, and some men do the same thing with women. The way of doing this (i.e. of kissing the yoni) should be known from kissing the mouth. When a man and woman lie down in an inverted order, i.e. with the head of the one towards the feet of the other and carry on this congress, it is called the "congress of a crow".'

For the sake of such things courtesans abandon men possessed of good qualities, liberal and clever, and become attached to low persons, such as slaves and elephant drivers. The Auparishtaka, or mouth congress, should never be done by a learned Brahman, by a minister that carries on the business of a state, or by a man of good reputation, because though the practice is allowed by the Shastras, there is no reason why it should be carried on, and need only be practised in particular cases. As for instance, the taste, and the strength, and the digestive qualities of the flesh of dogs are mentioned in works on medicine, but it does not therefore follow that it should be eaten by the wise. In the same way there are some men, some places and sometimes, with respect to which these practices can be made use of. A man should therefore pay regard to the place, to the time, and to the practice which is to be carried out, as also as to whether it is agreeable to his nature and to himself, and then he may or may not practice these things according to circumstances. But after all, these things being done secretly, and the mind of the man being fickle, how can it be known what any person will do at any particular time and for any particular purpose."

As far as oral sex goes, unfortunately in modern times, the practice of oral sex is becoming more and more lax. Women state that it's rare to find a man who enjoys performing oral sex on women; the same goes for men stating this about women. There are a lot of different reasons this may be attributed to modern times, partially because we tend to be a society of instant gratification. Oral sex takes time and performing it has to be done with passion and interest, otherwise the act is simply a waste.

Another reason why males don't go down on women as often as they should be; they are unsure of how to proceed once they are down there. Many men know where the clitoris is but they aren't sure what else goes on in the vagina in terms of discharge, menstrual cycles, etc. Every woman smells different and every woman tastes different and because of this, some men are surprised when they perform oral sex on a new woman. The best thing a woman can do for a man when he is performing oral sex is to let him know he is doing a good job and if he isn't, guide him in the right direction and tell him what you want.

A lot of the reason women don't participate in oral sex as much is the expectations some men have about women and pornography. A lot of men who watch a large amount of pornography assume that the women they are involved in will be able to do things such as repeated thrusting of the penis into the woman's throat or "deep throating'. Expectations like these are damaging to a relationship because they cause the men to over expect and the women to feel bad about themselves when they under achieve. Now, this isn't always the case, but this is becoming more and more frequent over the years.

Rachel Hughes

Chapter 6
Sex Positions

Sex isn't simply cut and dry, there are a bunch of different positions that people can do to enhance their sexual experience and allow for deeper penetration. The Kama Sutra lays out a bunch of different sexual positions. Going down the list, we will go over numerous sexual positions that will not only provide you with sexual satisfaction but also bring you and your lover closer together on a deep, intimate level.

The following positions are the ones we are going to go over:

Widely opened position

In order to perform this position, the woman should place a pillow under her head for comfort. Lying on her back, the man will kneel down in front of her and she will arch her back up, leaving her arms at her sides and placing her hands on his thighs. He will then insert himself inside her, gently moving up and down on. If his legs become tired, she can move her pelvis up and down. He can place his hands on either side of her back.

Yawning position

The yawning position requires the lady to lie on her back. Her legs are extended straight in front of her, resting the back of her legs on the front of the kneeling man's legs. While he is kneeling in front of her, he will insert himself inside her and will put his hands out. She will lace her fingers with his and using the leverage of her legs, he will lean forward to penetrate deeper inside of her.

Indrani

For this position, the woman lies on her back with her legs pulled up towards her chest. The man kneels in front of her, leaning his weight onto the back of her thighs. He will then place his hands on the outside of her knees. Placing a pillow underneath her head will help her stay comfortable. This position is intimate and with the right flexibility, couples can lock lips while performing this position.

Clasping position

The clasping position is most easily done with the male on the top. This position can be tricky to do and requires the right anatomy to have it done correctly; i.e., average to longer penises work best in this position. The woman will lay on her back, legs straight out in front of her, flat on the ground. The man will lay the exact same way on top of the woman, inserting himself inside her. This position is not meant for deep penetration but it's a wonderful position for intimacy as far as kissing and stroking one another. The roles can also be reversed where the man is on the bottom and the woman is on top.

Mares position

The mare's positon requires the woman to be on top, straddling the male. While straddling, the man is on his back, thrusting his pelvis upward into the woman. He can hold her hips or her arms, whichever he prefers. This position allows for deep penetration.

Rising position

The rising position is done by the woman laying on her back. She arches her back up in a wide "v" like position. This position is similar to previous positions except instead of the male thrusting into the woman, the woman thrusts her pelvis upward. She hangs onto the man's arms while he leans over her, almost as if in missionary position.

Pressed position

The pressed position is another position that allows for deep penetration. The woman lays on her back and pulls her knees up to her chest. The kneels in front of her and grabs her knees, she places her hands on his hips. This position gives the woman freedom to stimulate her clitoris or touch the male in different areas such as is chest, nipples, and abdomen.

Half pressed position

The half pressed position is a bit difficult to explain but incredibly pleasurable. This position requires the female to lay on her back, her right leg pulled up towards her chest. The male will kneel in front her, placing his left leg outside of her right leg and extending his right leg back behind him. The woman will take her left leg and rest it over the back of the male's right leg. She can place her hands on his torso or on her clitoris for added stimulation. From here, the male will thrust into the woman.

Splitting of a bamboo

For the splitting of the bamboo sex position, this requires the female to lay on her side, one leg stretched upward and the other straight out flat. The man will kneel in between her legs; one on either side of her pelvis. From here, she will rest her leg that is in the air on her lover's chest while he thrusts himself into her. This gives both parties a significant amount of contact making this position more intimate than others. The male can also use his hand to stimulate her clitoris or touch her breasts.

Fixing of a nail

The fixing of a nail sex position requires a bit more flexibility than others. Described best by Yvonne K. Fulbright, PhD, MSEd, a nationally known sex therapist and author of several books on sexuality, states that "Once she is lying on her back, her lover takes one leg up and moves her into a split, stretching her leg up vertically. As he kneels around her pelvis, he rests her foot against his forehead and begins to penetrate. She then alternates legs, placing her foot against his forehead and placing the first leg flat, and then repeating. This changes the angle of each thrust, with her lover's chest against the back of her thigh moving her up and down."

Crabs position

The crabs position is an interesting spin on the cowgirl position. This position requires the male to lay on his back while the female sits facing the male, placing a foot on either side of the male's head. He will grab onto her thighs with his hands and she can grab his shins with her hands. This position is also great for deep penetration and gives the male a great view of the woman's body and of the penetration. The couple can rock back and forth or the woman can hold herself up while the male thrusts himself upward, into her.

Packed position

The packed position is when the female extends her thighs and rests them each one on top of the other. The male can take her thighs in his arms and enter her while on his knees, kneeling.

Lotus-like position

The lotus like position is a highly sensual position, allowing both partners to be face to face with one another, embracing and kissing one another. The male will sit down, crossing his legs widely. The woman will sit in his lap, facing him and wrapping her legs around his back. While sitting down, she will lower herself onto his penis. This is also a deep penetration position and can be painful for men with larger penises. The woman can move up and down or back and forth while also getting clitoral stimulation from rubbing against the male's public region due to the positioning.

Turning position

Requiring a relative amount of physical strength from the male, this position has been referred to in modern times, quite accurately I might add, as "the helicopter". The man will insert himself inside the woman as if performing missionary position. From there, he will remain inside the woman while turning in a circle. Think of the woman as the body of the helicopter and the male as the top propeller for the helicopter. The penis is what is keeping this helicopter connected. This position appears to be intended more for show and experimentation than actual sexual pleasure.

Congress of a cow

The congress of a cow is actually an oral sex driven position that is a spin-off of the sixty-nine position (69). In this position, the male will lay on his side and the woman will lay on her side as well, facing him but at the opposite end. Her face should be facing his penis and his face should be facing her vagina. From here, the male will wrap his arms around the woman's pelvis and proceed to perform oral pleasure on the woman while the female performs oral pleasure on the male.

The visitor

The visitor is a position that can be done standing up if you both are the same height, or it can also be done with the woman's bottom resting on the edge of the table if the male is significantly taller than she is. In this position, the male will step closely to the female, embracing her as if to hug her and placing his hands on her lower back. She will the move one of her thighs in between his legs with her other leg still located on the outside of his legs. She will insert him inside of her and wrap her arms around his neck, gently moving herself up and down. This position works well if the male has a longer penis and if both individuals are the same height.

The toad

The toad, although not a very appealing name, is a deep penetrating sexual position that also allows for a great deal of intimacy. This position is initiated with the female laying on her back as if to perform the missionary position. Once on her back, the male will come at her, inserting himself inside her and stretching his legs out straight behind him. She will then pull her legs up higher and move her pelvis up and down while he is inside her. He can wrap his arms around her neck and she can reciprocate or grab his bottom. This sexual position is incredibly intimate and can also be relatively painful if the male has a longer penis so proceed gently at first.

Bandoleer

The bandoleer is similar to other sexual positions we have discussed, only a few different placements of the feet and hands make this position even more erotic. The female will lay on her back and pull her feet up to her chest. The male will kneel and insert himself inside her. She will place her feet on his pectoral muscles and he will cross his arms, placing each elbow on one of her knees and lifting her pelvis slightly. You can also place a pillow underneath her head for added comfort. The male will then thrust in and out slowly or in quick, short thrusts – whichever is preferred.

The slide

The slide is another sexual position that requires both individuals to lay on top of one another, laying out straight. This time though, the female is going to be on the top instead of the male. While the male is laying on his back, the female is going to lay on top of him in the same manner, wrapping her arms around his neck and lifting her pelvis up and down while he is inside her. Again, this is one of those positions that is best performed by people of similar length and with a meal who has a longer penis.

The rider

The rider is essentially the reverse cowgirl. The man will lay flat on his back and the woman will straddle him, facing towards his feet. She will place her hands on his ankles and use her knees to push herself up and down. The male can also help when she gets tired. This give the guy a great view while also giving the woman some control on penetration and speed.

The kneel

The kneel is an interesting position that is also a bit difficult to describe. To start, both lovers will be on their knees. The male will sit back on his calves, almost like kneeling. The woman will move in closer, straddling one of his kneeled legs and inserting him inside of her. He can wrap his arms around her back while she wraps her arms around his neck. Either he can thrust up and down or she can, it really depends on who is being the dominant force in the position.

The curled angel

The curled angel is a sweet sexual position that can be easily transitioned to after spooning. The position requires the male and female to both be lying on the sides, facing the same direction. The man will be behind the woman and the woman will pull her legs up to her chest, almost like the fetal position. The man will pull his legs up as well but will fold his legs with hers (his knees will be touching the back of her knees) and he will insert himself inside of her. He can lean up on his arm to get a better view of the woman and her breasts or he can lay down next to her and wrap his arm around her, embracing her.

The grip

One of the few positions formed with the male in the doggy style position, this position requires the male to bend over on his hands and knees over the woman. She will then thrust her pelvis into the air with her arms at her sides, thrusting him inside of her. From this position, you don't have to exert a lot of force but you are still able to get deep penetration and a great view. Either the male or female can thrust, rock back and forth or work together simultaneously.

Afternoon delight

Perfect for an afternoon quickie, this position requires the male to lay on his side and the woman to lay on her back, sitting on the male's penis. She will throw her legs over his hips while he thrusts in and out. This position is easily done on the bed and is another easily transition from the spooning position.

The eagle

A very popular position for many reasons. The eagle position has the female on her back with her legs spread open while the male inserts himself inside her from the front. He will grab her thighs and continue to thrust into her while her legs are spread open, giving him an amazing view of penetration, her clitoris and her breasts and face during intercourse. She also has the freedom to stimulate her clitoris if necessary to achieve climax.

The sphinx

An interesting rendition of the highly popular, doggy style position, the sphinx involved the woman laying on her stomach, sitting up on her elbows. She will then pull one leg up to her side and leave another leg stretched. The male will then put his weight on his hands, leaning over her with his legs stretched behind him, inserting himself inside her. He will then move up and down, thrusting gently. She can also help take some of the strain off of him but bouncing back onto him instead of having him do all the work.

The column

This position involved both parties standing up, the male behind the female. The male will then insert himself inside her from behind, wrapping his hands around her waist and placing them on her pubic region. She can place her hands over his or on a surface in front of her. The position is great for a couple who wants to have a quickie.

The clasp

This position requires either a relatively strong man or an incredibly light woman (or a combination of the two). The woman will wrap her legs around the man's waist, putting him inside of her. He will then hold her up, placing his arms on her bottom and lifting her up and down on his penis. If the weight is too much, this position can be modified by having her sit on a flat surface such as a tabletop or a counter – though the position will go by a different name if that's the case.

The seated ball

Another intimate sexual position, the seated ball requires the male to sit on his bottom, legs stretched out in front. The woman will then sit down in the man's lap, facing the same way. She will pull her legs closer to her chest, keeping them on the outside of his legs. She will then lean slightly forward and grab his ankles while he leans forward onto her back. This is an easy position for the woman to take control and guide the male into her on her terms, not his. This position requires a bit of strength and flexibility on the woman's part but don't let that keep you away from trying a modified version.

The perch

Using a chair as a perch, the man will sit on the chair (or stool) and have the woman sit down onto him, letting him inside her. She will be facing the same way he is, both of them placing their feet on the floor. He can wrap his arms around her waist and stimulate her clitoris or she can stimulate her clitoris while he holds her breasts. Though not a lot of visual stimulation, this position allows for a lot of touch on the male's part, giving him free rein over her body.

The plough

This position requires a bit of strength on both parties, along with a lower surface such as a bed. In the position, the woman will lay on the edge of the bed on her stomach with her legs straight out behind her, opened slightly for the male to walk in between. As the male walks in between, he will hold her legs up, taking some of the pressure off of her. He will lift her pelvis up so that he can put himself inside her while she balances on the bed on her arms or elbows. While the man is standing, holding her hips with her pelvis in the air, he will then begin thrusting (or ploughing) into her. The term comes from the way in which the man is holding the woman, almost as if he is plowing a field or using a push mower. This requires arm and abdominal strength and stamina from the woman as well as arm strength from the male.

The fan

This position is another spin off of the commonly known and incredibly loved doggy-style position. The woman will bend forward onto a stool, table, counter, or other hard surface that is lower than she is. From this position, she will arch her back, lifting her bottom higher in the air and giving the man a much better angle for entering her. He can place his hands on her bottom or wrap them around to stimulate her clitoris (even better if this is done during anal sex). This is called the fan because the man can thrust in a circular motion, similar to a fan.

The bridge

This sounds difficult because it is difficult. This can only be performed by a man who is capable of maintaining the weight of their female lover on their abdomen while also performing a backbend. This position requires the male the put himself in a backbend and have the woman climb onto him, placing her hands on his pectoral muscles and moving back and forth on his penis. For an added workout, the male could attempt to thrust in and out as well, though that is highly unlikely to be pleasurable. This position will be even more difficult if the female is short and unable to reach the ground while on top of the male, meaning the male will have to hold the entire weight of the woman while maintaining his back bend. Do not attempt this if you are unsure of your strength.

The crouching tiger

This sexual position is another form of reverse cowgirl. The male will lay on his back on the edge of the bed, letting his feet touch the floor. From here, the woman will climb onto him lap on reverse cowgirl position, pulling her feet up beside her and using them to move up and down as opposed to being on her knees. From this position she can stimulate either her own clitoris or fondle her lover's testicles. When her legs get tired, the male can take over and thrust while the woman lifts her pelvis slightly above his pelvis, giving him room to thrust. This position doesn't require must strength on the males side but it does require a bit of leg strength from the woman's side.

Attempting anal sex can be done with nearly all of these positions, the only thing to keep in mind is that both parties are in agreement on the activity. With anal sex, both individuals are at a higher risk for infection and injury so only attempt anal sex with someone you trust. Due to the high risk for infection, protection is encouraged to protect the male and the female; the male is protected from any diseases or bacteria that may become lodged in his urethra, while the female is protected from semen and possible bacteria on the male's penis.

Excessive lubrication needs to be used when performing anal sex as well, due to the high risk for tearing and abrasion. Even a small cut can become infected because of the high amount of bacteria in the area, so make sure the female is comfortable and not feeling any pain upon penetration. Listen to her signals and have her reassure you that she is comfortable.

Anal sex can be highly pleasurable for women when performed correctly and safely because of the access that the penis has to the g-spot through the rectum. During anal sex, the penis will rub over the g-spot through the tissue of the rectum, creating an incredibly arousing sensation that some woman can even climax over. Our rectum has a large amount of nerves – more than we realize, which is why it can be so pleasurable when used for intercourse. Unfortunately, though, we can't argue with anatomy and our anus was designed as an exit as opposed to an entrance so make sure the exit is clear before attempting anal sex.

Chapter 7
Charms, Aphrodisiacs, Artificial Membranes And Sex Toys

Charms; meaning certain ways in which one can lure or charm an individual into desire, were commonly used and practiced with in Ancient Indian times. Modern day spells and recipes that are focused on aphrodisiac like qualities are seen as far-fetched, though some claim they are effective. The Kama Sutra laid out a large number of recipes (or charms) that focused on the following types of spells:

- "Affection for her husband

- Desire of lawful progeny

- Want of opportunity

- Anger at being addressed by the man too familiarly

- Difference in rank of life

- Want of certainty on account of the man being devoted travelling

- Thinking that the man may be attached to some other person

- Fear of the man's not keeping his intentions secret

- Thinking that the man is too devoted to his friends, and has too great a regard for them

- The apprehension that he is not in earnest

- Bashfulness on account of his being an illustrious man

- Fear on account of his being powerful, or possessed of too impetuous passion, in the case of the deer woman

- Bashfulness on account of his being too clever

- The thought of having once lived with him on friendly terms only

- Contempt of his want of knowledge of the world

- Distrust of his low character

- Disgust at his want of perception of her love for him

- In the case of an elephant woman, the thought that he is a hare man, or a man of weak passion

- Compassion lest anything should befall him on account of his passion

- Despair at her own imperfections

- Fear of discovery

- Disillusion at seeing his grey hair or shabby appearance

- Fear that he may be employed by her husband to test her chastity

- The thought that he has too much regard for morality"

For the sake of entertainment and history, the following recipes were considered to be effective in winning over desirable individuals. Some of these recipes are seen more as experiment's or placebo effect as opposed to actual reactions, but in ancient times these effects felt real. In fact, some of these recipes contain actual aphrodisiac items that can create arousal in certain individuals. Keep in mind "lingam" is the male penis and when you see Vatsyayana referring to deer women or bull man, these are in relation to the classifications earlier on in the book. The following recipes and experiments are as follows:

- "The armlet' (Valaya) should be of the same size as the lingam, and should have its outer surface made rough with globules.

- 'The couple' (Sanghati) is formed of two armlets

- 'The bracelet' (Chudaka, cudaka) is made by joining three or more armlets, until they come up to the required length of the lingam.

- 'The single bracelet' is formed by wrapping a single wire around the lingam, according to its dimensions.

- The Kantuka or Jalaka is a tube open at both ends, with a hole through it, outwardly rough and studded with soft globules, and made to fit the side of the yoni, and tied to the waist.When such a thing cannot be obtained, then a tube made of the wood apple, or tubular stalk of the bottle gourd, or a reed made soft with oil and extracts of plants, and tied to the waist with strings, may be made use of, as also a row of soft pieces of wood tied together.

The above are the things that can be used in connection with or in the place of the lingam.

The people of the southern countries think that true sexual pleasure cannot be obtained without perforating the lingam, and they therefore cause it to be pierced like the lobes of the ears of an infant pierced for earrings.

Now, when a young man perforates his lingam he should pierce it with a sharp instrument, and then stand in water so long as the blood continues to flow. At night, he should engage in sexual intercourse, even with vigour, so as to clean the hole. After this he should continue to wash the hole with decoctions, and increase the size by putting into it small pieces of cane, and the wrightia antidysenterica, and thus gradually enlarging the orifice. It may also be washed with liquorice mixed with honey, and the size of the hole increased by the fruit stalks of the simapatra plant. The hole should also be anointed with a small quantity of oil.

In the hole made in the lingam a man may put Apadravyas of various forms, such as the 'round', the 'round on one side', the 'wooden mortar', the 'flower', the 'armlet', the 'bone of the heron', the 'goad of the elephant', the 'collection of eight balls', the 'lock of hair', the 'place where four roads meet', and other things named according to their forms and means of using them. All these Apadravyas should be rough on the outside according to their requirements.

The ways of enlarging the lingam must be now related.

When a man wishes to enlarge his lingam, he should rub it with the bristles of certain insects that live in trees, and then, after rubbing it for ten nights with oils, he should again rub it with the bristles as before. By continuing to do this a swelling will be gradually produced in the lingam, and he should then lie on a cot, and cause his lingam to hang down through a hole in the cot. After this he should take away all the pain from the swelling by using cool concoctions. The swelling, which is called 'Suka', and is often brought about among the people of the Dravida country, lasts for life.

If the lingam is rubbed with the following things, the plant physalis flexuosa, the shavara-kandaka plant, the jalasuka plant, the fruit of the egg plant, the butter of a she buffalo, the hastri-charma plant, and the juice of the vajrarasa plant, a swelling lasting for one month will be produced.

By rubbing it with oil boiled in the concoctions of the above things, the same effect will be produced, but lasting for six months.

The enlargement of the lingam is also effected by rubbing it or moistening it with oil boiled on a moderate fire along with the seeds of the pomegranate, and the cucumber, the juices of the valuka plant, the hastri-charma plant, and the eggplant.

In addition to the above, other means may be learnt from experienced and confidential persons.

The miscellaneous experiments and recipes are as follows:

If a man mixes the powder of the milk hedge plant, and the kantaka plant with the excrement of a monkey and the powdered root of the lanjalika plant, and throws this mixture on a woman, she will not love anybody else afterwards.

If a man thickens the juice of the fruits of the cassia fistula, and the eugenia jambolana by mixing them with the powder of the soma plant, the vernonia anthelmintica, the eclipta prostata, and the lohopa-jihirka, and applies this composition to the yoni of a woman, and then has sexual intercourse with her, his love for her will be destroyed.

The same effect is produced if a man has connection with a woman who has bathed in the buttermilk of a she-buffalo mixed with the powders of the gopalika plant, the banu-padika plant and the yellow amaranth.

An ointment made of the flowers of the nauclea cadamba, the hog plum, and the eugenia jambolana, and used by a woman, causes her to be disliked by her husband.

Garlands made of the above flowers, when worn by the woman, produce the same effect.

An ointment made of the fruit of the asteracantha longifolia (kokilaksha) will contract the yoni of a Hastini or Elephant woman, and this contraction lasts for one night.

An ointment made by pounding the roots of the nelumbrium speciosum, and of the blue lotus, and the powder of the plant physalis flexuosa mixed with ghee and honey, will enlarge the yoni of the Mrigi or Deer woman.

An ointment made of the fruit of the emblica myrabolans soaked in the milky juice of the milk hedge plant, of the soma plant, the calotropis gigantea, and the juice of the fruit of the vernonia anthelmintica, will make the hair white.

The juice of the roots of the madayantaka plant, the yellow amaranth, the anjanika plant, the clitoria ternateea, and the shlakshnaparin plant, used as a lotion, will make the hair grow.

An ointment made by boiling the above roots in oil, and rubbed in, will make the hair black, and will also gradually restore hair that has fallen off.

If lac is saturated seven times in the sweat of the testicle of a white horse, and applied to a red lip, the lip will become white.

The colour of the lips can be regained by means of the madayantika and other plants mentioned above.

A woman who hears a man playing on a reed pipe which has been dressed with the juices of the bahupadika plant, the tabernamontana coronaria, the costus speciosus or arabicus, the pinus deodora, the euphorbia antiquorum, the vajra and the kantaka plant, becomes his slave.

If food be mixed with the fruit of the thorn apple (dathura) it causes intoxication.

If water be mixed with oil and the ashes of any kind of grass except the kusha grass, it becomes the colour of milk.

If yellow myrabolans, the hog plum, the shrawana plant, and the priyangu plant be all pounded together, and applied to iron pots, these pots become red.

If a lamp, trimmed with oil extracted from the shrawana and priyangu plants, its wick being made of cloth and the slough of the skins of snakes, is lighted, and long pieces of wood placed near it, those pieces of wood will resemble so many snakes.

Drinking the milk of a white cow who has a white calf at her foot is auspicious, produces fame, and preserves life.

The blessings of venerable Brahmans, well propitiated, have the same effect.

There are also some verses in conclusion:

'Thus have I written in a few words the "Science of love", after reading the texts of ancient authors, and following the ways of enjoyment mentioned in them.'

'He who is acquainted with the true principles of this science pays regard to Dharma, Artha, Kama, and to his own experiences, as well as to the teachings of others, and does not act simply on the dictates of his own desire. As for the errors in the science of love which I have mentioned in this work, on my own authority as an author, I have, immediately after mentioning them, carefully censured and prohibited them.'

'An act is never looked upon with indulgence for the simple reason that it is authorised by the science, because it ought to be remembered that it is the intention of the science, that the rules which it contains should only be acted upon in particular cases. After reading and considering the works of Babhravya and other ancient authors, and thinking over the meaning of the rules given by them, the Kama Sutra was composed, according to the precepts of Holy Writ, for the benefit of the world, by Vatsyayana, while leading the life of a religious student, and wholly engaged in the contemplation of the Deity.'

'This work is not intended to be used merely as an instrument for satisfying our desires. A person, acquainted with the true principles of this science, and who preserves his Dharma, Artha, and Kama, and has regard for the practices of the people, is sure to obtain the mastery over his senses. 'In short, an intelligent and prudent person, attending to Dharma and Artha, and attending to Kama also, without becoming the slave of his passions, obtains success in everything that he may undertake.'

An ointment made of the tabernamontana coronaria, the costus speciosus or arabicus, and the flacourtia cataphracta, can be used as an unguent of adornment.

If a fine powder is made of the above plants, and applied to the wick of a lamp, which is made to burn with the oil of blue vitrol, the black pigment or lamp black produced therefrom, when applied to the eyelashes, has the effect of making a person look lovely.

The oil of the hogweed, the echites putescens, the sarina plant, the yellow amaranth, and the leaf of the nymphae, if applied to the body, has the same effect. A black pigment from the same plants produces a similar effect.

By eating the powder of the nelumbrium speciosum, the blue lotus, and the mesna roxburghii, with ghee and honey, a man becomes lovely in the eyes of others.

The above things, together with the tabernamontana coronaria, and the xanthochymus pictorius, if used as an ointment, produce the same results.

If the bone of a peacock or of a hyena be covered with gold, and tied on the right hand, it makes a man lovely in the eyes of other people.

In the same way, if a bead, made of the seed of the jujube, or of the conch shell, be enchanted by the incantations mentioned in the Atharvana Veda, or by the incantations of those well skilled in the science of magic, and tied on the hand, it produces the same result as described above.

When a female attendant arrives at the age of puberty, her master should keep her secluded, and when men ardently desire her on account of her seclusion, and on account of the difficulty of approaching her, he should then bestow her hand on such a person as may endow her with wealth and happiness. This is a means of increasing the loveliness of a person in the eyes of others.

In the same way, when the daughter of a courtesan arrives at the age of puberty, the mother should get together a lot of young men of the same age, disposition, and knowledge as her daughter, and tell them that she would give her in marriage to the person who would give her presents of a particular kind.

After this the daughter should be kept in seclusion as far as possible, and the mother should give her in marriage to the man who may be ready to give her the presents agreed upon. If the mother is unable to get so much out of the man, she should show some of her own things as having been given to the daughter by the bridegroom.

Or the mother may allow her daughter to be married to the man privately, as if she was ignorant of the whole affair, and then pretending that it has come to her knowledge, she may give her consent to the union.

The daughter, too, should make herself attractive to the sons of wealthy citizens, unknown to her mother, and make them attached to her, and for this purpose should meet them at the time of learning to sing, and in places where music is played, and at the houses of other people, and then request her mother, through a female friend, or servant, to be allowed to unite herself to the man who is most agreeable to her.

When the daughter of a courtesan is thus given to a man, the ties of marriage should be observed for one year, and after that she may do what she likes. But even after the end of the year, when otherwise engaged, if she should be now and then invited by her first husband to come and see him, she should put aside her present gain, and go to him for the night.

Such is the mode of temporary marriage among courtesans, and of increasing their loveliness, and their value in the eyes of others. What has been said about them should also be understood to apply to the daughters of dancing women, whose mothers should give them only to such persons as are likely to become useful to them in various ways. Thus end the ways of making oneself lovely in the eyes of others.

If a man, after anointing his lingam with a mixture of the powders of the white thorn apple, the long pepper and, the black pepper, and honey, engages in sexual union with a woman, he makes her subject to his will.

The application of a mixture of the leaf of the plant vatodbhranta, of the flowers thrown on a human corpse when carried out to be burnt, and the powder of the bones of the peacock, and of the jiwanjiva bird produces the same effect.

The remains of a kite who has died a natural death, ground into powder, and mixed with cowach and honey, has also the same effect.

Anointing oneself with an ointment made of the plant emblica myrabolans has the power of subjecting women to one's will.

If a man cuts into small pieces the sprouts of the vajnasunhi plant, and dips them into a mixture of red arsenic and sulphur, and then dries them seven times, and applies this powder mixed with honey to his lingam, he can subjugate a woman to his will directly that he has had sexual union with her, or if, by burning these very sprouts at night and looking at the smoke, he sees a golden moon behind, he will then be successful with any woman; or if he throws some of the powder of these same sprouts mixed with the excrement of a monkey upon a maiden, she will not be given in marriage to anybody else.

If pieces of the arris root are dressed with the oil of the mango, and placed for six months in a hole made in the trunk of the sisu tree, and are then taken out and made up into an ointment, and applied to the lingam, this is said to serve as the means of subjugating women.

If the bone of a camel is dipped into the juice of the plant eclipta prostata, and then burnt, and the black pigment produced from its ashes is placed in a box also made of the bone of a camel, and applied together with antimony to the eye lashes with a pencil also made of the bone of a camel, then that pigment is said to be very pure, and wholesome for the eyes, and serves as a means of subjugating others to the person who uses it. The same effect can be produced by black pigment made of the bones of hawks, vultures, and peacocks. Thus end the ways of subjugating others to one's own will.

Now the means of increasing sexual vigour are as follows

A man obtains sexual vigour by drinking milk mixed with sugar, the root of the uchchata plant, the piper chaba, and liquorice.

Drinking milk, mixed with sugar, and having the testicle of a ram or a goat boiled in it, is also productive of vigour.

The drinking of the juice of the hedysarum gangeticum, the kuili, and the kshirika plant mixed with milk, produces the same effect.

The seed of the long pepper along with the seeds of the sanseviera roxburghiana, and the hedysarum gangeticum plant, all pounded together, and mixed with milk, is productive of a similar result.

According to ancient authors, if a man pounds the seeds or roots of the trapa bispinosa, the kasurika, the tuscan jasmine, and liquorice, together with the kshirakapoli (a kind of onion), and puts the powder into milk mixed with sugar and ghee, and having boiled the whole mixture on a moderate fire, drinks the paste so formed, he will be able to enjoy innumerable women.

In the same way, if a man mixes rice with the eggs of the sparrow, and having boiled this in milk, adds to it ghee and honey, and drinks as much of it as necessary, this will produce the same effect.

If a man takes the outer covering of sesamum seeds, and soaks them with the eggs of sparrows, and then, having boiled them in milk, mixed with sugar and ghee, along with the fruits of the trapa bispinosa and the kasurika plant, and adding to it the flour of wheat and beans, and then drinks this composition, he is said to be able to enjoy many women.

If ghee, honey, sugar and licorice in equal quantities, the juice of the fennel plant, and milk are mixed together, this nectar-like composition is said to be holy, and provocative of sexual vigor, a preservative of life, and sweet to the taste.

The drinking of a paste composed of the asparagus racemosus, the shvadaushtra plant, the guduchi plant, the long pepper, and licorice, boiled in milk, honey, and ghee, in the spring, is said to have the same effect as the above.

Boiling the asparagus racemosus, and the shvadaushtra plant, along with the pounded fruits of the premna spinose in water, and drinking the same, is said to act in the same way.

Drinking boiled ghee, or clarified butter, in the morning during the spring season, is said to be beneficial to health and strength and agreeable to the taste.

If the powder of the seed of the shvadaushtra plant and the flower of barley are mixed together in equal parts, and a portion of it, i.e. two palas in weight, is eaten every morning on getting up, it has the same effect as the preceding recipe."

As you can probably see, most of these recipes are outrageous and foolish, though some state that the effectiveness of them cannot be compared. Modern day medicine doesn't offer much of an option for men looking to enlarge the size of their penis, so recipes such as these give hope to men who aren't as well-endowed as others and who are ashamed.

Now, switching back over to modern times, there are a lot of modern day aphrodisiacs and toys that can be used to spice up the sex life in the bedroom outside of outrageous and difficult concoctions. Some proven aphrodisiac foods are:

Oysters – who would have thought? They contain high amounts of zinc that help with fertility along with a wide range of amino acids that are said to aid in the arousal of the individual.

Chili peppers are another unexpected aphrodisiac, they are said to be the food of love because of their bright, red color. This food also mimics how one feels when aroused by speeding up the heart rate and causing you to perspire; both of which happen when one is aroused.

Avocado is another aphrodisiac due to the high amounts of Vitamin E. It is unclear how or when the arousal occurs with this food but the rich yet mild taste makes it easily morphed to taste like nearly anything it's added to.

We all know about the sexual effects of chocolate. Many have said that consuming chocolate actually gives people the feeling of being in love. Chocolate releases dopamine into the body, creating a euphoric sensation upon consumption. This is often why chocolate is used in the bedroom during foreplay as a syrup or a chocolate powder.

Bananas are said to be aphrodisiacs as well due to the triggering of testosterone production in males and the elevation of energy due to the high amounts of potassium and Vitamin B. Not only is this food healthy for you, it can also be consumed a variety of different ways.

Another fun ingredient to use in the bedroom that is also arousing is whipped cream. We aren't talking about the cheaper, zero calorie whipped cream either. You want the rich, real whipped cream that you either make yourself or purchase from your local grocer.

Pine nuts and pumpkin seeds are surprising aphrodisiacs as well. Both high in vitamins and minerals that aid in sexual functioning such as zinc and magnesium, these nuts are easily incorporated into a variety of different recipes due to their milk flavors.

Among other aphrodisiac foods are honey, arugula, watermelon, coffee, figs, strawberries, artichokes, chai tea, cherries, pomegranate, red wine, salmon, walnuts, and vanilla.

Moving on to sex toys; today there exists more sex toys and variety than ever before. With the emergence of extreme, lifestyle sex toys in the form of robotic like women that not only move in sexual motions but also speak and have flesh like skin covering them. Some men keep these robots in their home as replacements to women, though these are extreme cases. More regular sex toys involve a variety of different items like the "cock ring".

This ring can be purchased as a one-time use ring or multiple use. Some of the rings are simply made to squeeze the male penis to keep more blood in the shaft which is especially helpful for men who have difficulty maintaining an erection. The ring helps to keep blood in the shaft and can also vibrate if the vibrating model is chosen. When the ring vibrates, the women can feel it when the male is inside of her adding extra sensation to the act of intercourse. Aside from aiding in the sustainment of an erection, these rings also give the man more sensation because of the heightened blood flow to his penis.

Dildos and vibrators can be used by both men and women during sexual intercourse. Dildos don't normally vibrate but they simulate the shape and feel of a real life penis. Vibrators can be small or shaped like a male penis while also having the option to vibrate or rotate. Some of these toys have grooves, notches and lumps on them for added sensations. Men can insert these items into women either vaginally or anally during foreplay or intercourse and women can insert these into the male anally during intercourse if he desires. These toys are great when the male isn't in the mood for intercourse because he can still help the woman climax by inserting the dildo or vibrator inside of her.

Another male toy is the prostate plug; it's a butt plug that is inserted into the male anally and intended to touch or rub against his prostate during intercourse or masturbation which can be highly pleasurable. Some of these prostate plugs even vibrate, creating a nearly unbearable euphoria. Butt plugs can also be used by women to help loosen the anus for penetration or longer ones can be inserted to touch the g-spot through the colon during intercourse. One thing to be careful with is making sure that what you are using is actually intended to be inserted anally.

Devices and toys that are created to be inserted anally come with a safety type guard that prevents them from being sucked up into your anus. Because your rectum is an exit rather than an entrance, it acts as a vacuum when anything foreign is inserted (which is why you are able to hold in your feces if you aren't near a bathroom). Muscle memory will assume that the foreign object is feces and will suck it back up into the rectum, causing a dangerous and potentially lethal situation if damage or tearing occurs. Only insert anally if it says it can be inserted anally.

More items can be used such as costumes and different types of bondage items like whips, handcuffs, gag balls, collars, edibles, etc. Those types of items are generally practiced by experienced couples who enjoy bondage and not by people who are unfamiliar or put off by bondage type attire.

Conclusion

After reading this book, I hope you were able to gain an amazing understanding of past and current sexual activities along with a variety of different ways to spice up your own sex life and enjoy you and your lover on a more intimate and sensual level. Sex can be as intimate or as shallow as you make it however, meaningful and passionate sex is almost always preferred. With this book you should be able to understand the initial purpose of the Kama Sutra and the principles that surrounded it.

The book gives the readers different types of kissing, behaviors, sexual positions and other techniques that can help us to become better lovers and learn more about one another sexually. One of the biggest issues in today's relationships is that people aren't exploring each other's bodies the way they used to. In Indian times, sex and the body was something to celebrate and enjoy together and explore. Simply speaking of your lover's body would get one aroused. In modern times, we are so quick to look the other way when we see something we don't like instead of looking at ways to like it.

With this book, I hope you are able to enter the bedroom with confidence to please your loved one and the willingness to do whatever it takes; and I hope they feel the same way. The Kama Sutra was right when it spoke of finding someone who is compatible with you anatomically and attitude wise. Someone who has a high sex drive isn't going to mesh well with someone who a has a low sex drive. You may be able to make it work on an emotional level but on a physical and sexual level, your relationship may fall short.

Granted, sex isn't everything in a relationship but it means more to some people in a relationship than it does to others so choose your lover wisely. This book should have also shown you different ways in which woman may have seen you in the past and in the future; same goes for woman and how men view them. In modern times, we don't much care for the way people see us but in ancient times, your reputation was everything. This book can be an eye opener to how some of your current behaviors may have been seen in ancient times – whether that affects you or not is your own accord.

Aside from many asinine doings involved in recipes, spells and charms, there were was also a lot of educational and interesting information on aphrodisiac foods and which ones work the best. Some people might not even realize the large amount of foods that can actually be arousing to certain individuals. We all have our own things that arouse us – scribble that in on the aphrodisiac section.

This book also gave you a great insight on different types of sexual positions that are spinoffs of some of the most well-known sexual positions that we all know so well. One of the biggest reasons individuals are unsatisfied with their sex life is due to redundancy and repetition. As humans, we naturally get tired of things; some of us more quickly than others. It is my hope that with this book, you can quickly turn to the different pages and find something new for you to try to spice up you sex life.

It is very easy to slip into a life of routine which isn't necessarily a bad thing, unless it has to do with your sex life and learning. Two things you should never stop doing: learning and experimenting in the bedroom. After all is said and done, take the knowledge you have received from this book as either a grain of salt or as your new sexual bible. Hope you enjoyed!

If you received value from this book, then I would like to ask you for a favor. Would you be kind enough to leave a review for this book on Amazon?

Thank you so much!

Rachel Hughes

Made in the USA
Middletown, DE
30 June 2019